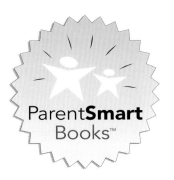

ParentSmart Books™

Medical Emergencies & Childhood Illnesses

Includes Your Child's Personal Health Journal

Penny A. Shore

with

William Sears, M.D.

Canadian Cataloguing in Publication Data

Shore, Penny A.
Medical emergencies & childhood illnesses

ISBN 1-896833-18-7

Includes index. 1. Pediatric emergencies - Popular works. 2. Children - Diseases. I. Sears, William, M.D.
II. Title. III. Title: Medical emergencies and childhood illnesses. IV. Series: Shore, Penny A.
Parent**Smart** Books.

RJ61.S52 2002   618.98'0025   C2001-901957-2

Published by The Parent Kit Corporation
2 Bloor Street West, Suite 1720
Toronto, Ontario M4W 3E2

Printed in Canada, by St. Joseph Printing Ltd.
First printing November 2001

1 2 3 4 5   05 04 03 02 01

ParentSmart Books
introduction to the series

Parenting has been my passion ever since the day my first child was born. This was, without doubt, an exhilarating and exciting event. However, it didn't take long to realize that with the birth of our child, we were taking on one of the most important jobs in life – and one for which we hadn't taken a training course. Furthermore, the baby didn't come with an instruction manual!

Now, my children have grown into happy, successful young adults and although my job is educational publishing, I have always considered parenting to be my most satisfying career. About four years ago, it occurred to me that I could combine my passion for parenting with my publishing experience. The idea was to produce a series of books designed to give new parents the very help and guidance I was looking for as a new parent. To develop the content, four of the world's leading parenting authorities were recruited to join me in establishing The International Advisory Council on Parenting. The members are; Penelope Leach, Ph.D., Otto Weininger, Ph.D., William Sears, M.D. and Martha Sears, R.N. The result of our combined efforts is the Parent**Smart** book series.

Despite the daily challenges faced by parents, there is probably no job in the world that matches parenting in terms of personal fulfillment and truly wonderful fringe benefits.

Parents who are properly prepared with the right tools and skills will have less stress and are likely to be more effective. That's why each book in the Parent**Smart** book series deals with one particular aspect of parenting. Taken together, the first six books in the series combine to provide a virtual "Parenting 101" course.

These books are unique in many ways. They provide you with a combination of expert information, interactive exercises and journals where you can record important information about your child. By having the full series available in your home, you will have easy access to the knowledge and support you will need to confidently handle most parenting situations.

There is another feature of the Parent**Smart** series that is very special. The experts don't necessarily agree on all parenting issues, and this can be confusing to parents who want their child to benefit from the best advice. We resolved this by having all members of The International Advisory Council on Parenting approve and come to consensus on the content.

A complete list of the other titles in this series, and a description of their contents, can be found at the back of this book. Parent**Smart** books are also a good refresher and primer for new grandparents, child caretakers and others in your extended family who will interact with your child.

Try to complete the questionnaires and exercises when you can. This will help you and your parenting partner to have a basis for communicating on the important issues and to be a better parenting team. The journals will provide records that you can enjoy and share with your children when they are older. "Tips and Techniques" are highlighted in the book to help you make immediate use of your new skills in every day situations.

I hope this book will raise your awareness about important parenting issues and give you the confidence to be a more effective and nurturing parent. Nothing can match the pleasure and happiness of seeing your children grow into fulfilled adults who are getting the best from their lives and whose friendship you cherish.

It has now been well-established that investing in your child's first three years will pay dividends in determining his or her future development. So, good luck with this stage and may your parenting adventure be one of the most rewarding experiences of your lifetime.

Penny Shore

dedication

To Joan, Eric, Jay and Amanda —
from whom I continue to learn.

your emergency kit

The following is a list of suggested materials that you should have available in an emergency:

- acetaminophen (liquid, suppositories or chewable form for older children)
- adhesive tape
- alcohol swabs
- antibiotic ointment
- antiseptic solution
- Band-Aids
- cotton balls
- cotton-tip applicators
- flashlight
- gauze pads (nonstick)
- gloves (sterile latex)
- hydrogen peroxide
- instant ice packs
- ipecac syrup
- nasal aspirator
- saline nose drops or saline nasal spray
- scissors with blunt ends
- steri-strips (butterfly bandages)
- thermometer
- tweezers with blunt ends

Medical Emergencies & Childhood Illnesses

Table of Contents

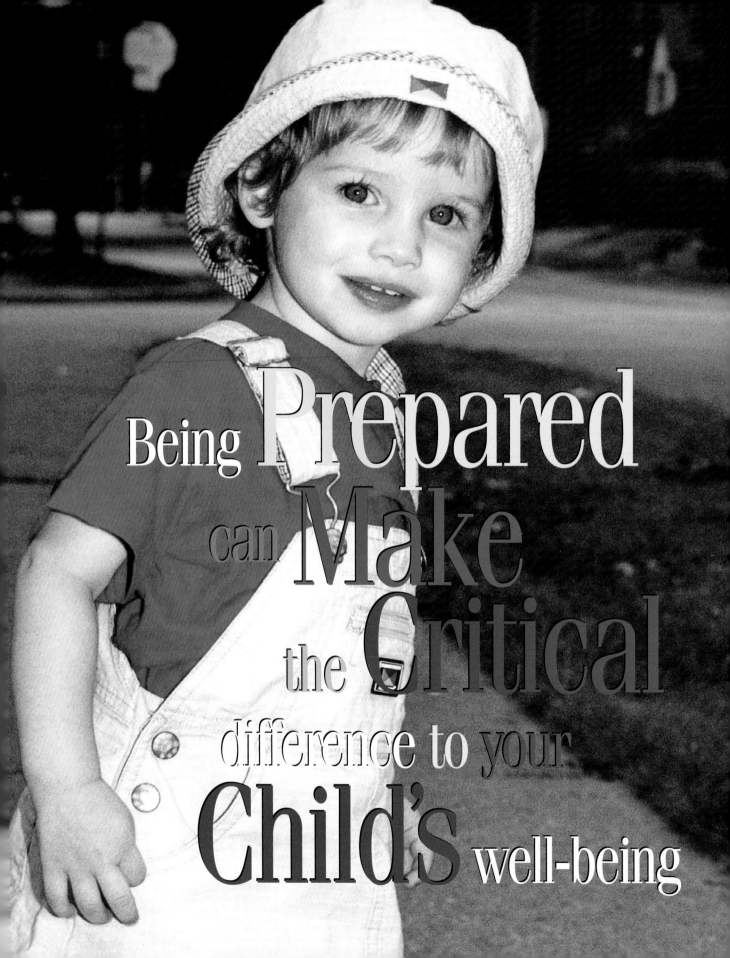

Being **Prepared** can **Make** the **Critical** difference to your **Child's** well-being

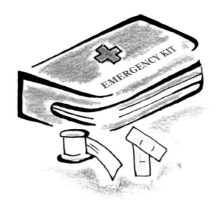

medical emergencies

introduction

No matter how carefully you watch or care for your child, medical emergencies **can** arise. In the event that they do, being prepared can make the critical difference to your child's well-being.

That's why you would be well advised to take a course in first aid, including training in cardiopulmonary resuscitation (CPR), and to ensure that your child's caregivers have this training as well. The procedures described in this book cannot provide a suitable substitute for getting the training you need.

Be prepared. Clearly post in your home the names and numbers of emergency personnel in your area, as well as filling them in on page 75 of this book. Include paramedics, the local poison control center, the police department, the fire department, the nearest major hospital and your child's doctor. Keep these numbers current, and teach your children their importance and where they can find them.

Keep this book in an accessible spot and tell each of your child's caregivers where it is kept. Familiarize yourself with the information in this book before you need it, so that you can access it quickly in an emergency. Again, it is important to realize that we're only providing you with basic information – always get professional help when you need it. Trust your instincts. In some cases, emergencies are clear-cut and immediate action is required. Others may not be so obvious. If you have any doubt and you think you may be facing an emergency, err on the side of caution. Call emergency personnel right away.

In case follow-up treatment is necessary after you administer first aid, always call your doctor (except in very minor situations) as an extra cautionary measure – even if your child seems fine.

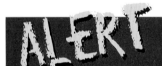 **in case of a severe medical emergency**

A child with severe allergies or a chronic medical condition (such as food, insect and drug allergies, or diabetes or asthma), which may influence the action taken in an emergency situation, should always wear medical identification – like a medical alert bracelet – to warn all caregivers of the child's condition. Also, some medical conditions – for example, insect allergies – require special equipment or medications. Make sure your child is always carrying the appropriate medications in case of an emergency.

acetaminophen dosage guide

Many of the treatments in this book suggest administering acetaminophen. The suggested dosages are intended as a guide for safely administering acetaminophen to your baby or child. As a rule, it is safe to give 7 milligrams of acetaminophen per pound of body weight every 4 hours. If you measure your child's body weight in kilograms, as a rule it is safe to give 10 to a maximum of 15 mg per kilogram of body weight every 4 hours. (See chart below for dosages.) **Pay careful attention to the form of acetaminophen you are giving your child, as different forms (for example, drops and syrup) often come in different concentrations.**

Dosages recommended can be given every 4 hours, but you should not give more than 5 doses in 24 hours.

Age	0-3 months	4-11 months	12-23 months	2-3 years
Weight	6-11 lbs.	12-17 lbs.	18-23 lbs.	24-35 lbs.
	(3-5 kg)	(5.5-8 kg)	(8-10.5 kg)	(10.5-16 kg)
Dosage	40-80 mg	80-120 mg	120-160 mg	160-240 mg

Note: If acetaminophen is given for fever, dressing the child lightly while preventing shivering and assuring adequate fluid intake is also very important. Baths and alcohol friction rubs are not recommended. The administration of ASA (acetylsalicylic acid) is not recommended in feverish children and youth. The reason for this is that, if the fever is due to chicken pox, flu or other viral infections, taking ASA increases the risk of Reye's Syndrome, a serious illness, which could affect the child's liver and the brain.

essential steps to take
in all emergency situations

- Always be calm in an emergency, as your child will take your cue. If you panic, the child is likely to panic as well, and this may make rescue procedures more difficult or life threatening.

- Always wash your hands thoroughly before beginning any treatment to prevent infection.

- Whenever blood is involved in an injury, try to wear sterile latex gloves to prevent the spread of infectious diseases transmittable by blood.

- Any time a child has been injured, you should be sure to assess the situation, so that you know exactly how serious it is. Here are a few things that you should always check.

- Check the ABC's – Airway, Breathing, Circulation (pulse). By doing this, you will be able to tell if the heart and lungs are functioning and keeping the child alive, or whether the child needs assistance until medical help arrives.

  - Look in the child's mouth to determine if there is anything that you can see that is obstructing the airway. Carefully remove any obstruction that you can see, but do not blindly poke around and push it further into the airway or lungs. If you suspect that the child's airway is blocked, *see Choking on page 32.*

  - Check the child's breathing by looking at the chest to see if it's rising and falling. Listen with your ear at the child's mouth for sounds of breathing, and feel for air on your ear. If the child is not breathing but has a pulse, *see Artificial Respiration on page 16.*

- For a baby (under one year), check the pulse by pressing gently with the fingertips of your hand on the inside of the baby's upper arm between the elbow and shoulder. If there is no pulse, *see CPR on page 28.*

- For a child (over one year), check the pulse by placing the fingertips of your hand (but not your thumb) on the large artery on the side of the child's neck. If there is no pulse, *see CPR on page 30.*

- After you check the ABC's, check for bleeding, poisoning, shock or broken bones. Treat appropriately until medical personnel arrives.

- You should also try to determine if the child could have a head, neck or back injury. Look for signs – for example, a stool or chair that the child may have fallen from, if it is positioned at the bottom of a flight of stairs.

- Do not move a child if there is a possibility of a back or neck injury, as doing so could cause further serious damage. Once you have assessed the situation, you will be able to advise any medical personnel who arrive on the scene what the child's status is.

- Whenever a child has been seriously injured, stopped breathing or lost his pulse, you should look for signs of shock once you have the immediate symptoms under control. If symptoms of shock are present, treat the child for shock. *See Shock on page 45.*

- Dial 911 or another emergency number when you need emergency medical help. Don't delay.

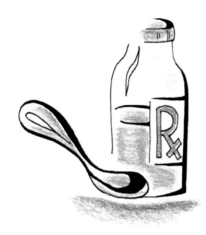

procedures for medical emergencies

On the following pages you will find a quick reference guide to general advice on how to handle common childhood medical emergencies.

Always try to remain calm as you assess the situation and be certain to call for medical help immediately if the situation seems beyond your capacity to deal with it, or life threatening.

NOTE: It is important to remember that this book will provide you with basic information only — always consult with your doctor if you are concerned.

allergic reaction, severe
(caused by insect bites, medication or food)
anaphylactic shock

Procedure

- **Call for medical emergency attention immediately.**

- **Symptoms:** weakness; difficulty breathing; wheezing; hives-like rash; severe itching; pale or blue skin; dizziness; anxiety; severe swelling at site of sting, or of hands and eyelids; stomach cramps and nausea; seizures or convulsions.

- Check the child's airway, breathing and circulation (pulse). If the child is not breathing or has no pulse, *see Artificial Respiration on page 16, or CPR on page 28.*

1. If you have had previous experience with allergies and your child and you have adrenaline (Epipen or Anakit), administer it immediately. With anaphylactic shock, every minute counts.

2. Lay the child on a flat surface, like a table or floor. Do not elevate the head if the child is having trouble breathing.

3. Speak to and act reassuringly with the child.

4. In case of vomiting, put the child on his side.

5. If the child has difficulty breathing, let him sit up.

6. Do not give the child any food, drink or medication by mouth.

7. Elevate the child's feet with a pillow or rolled-up blanket.

8. Keep the child warm.

Note: A child with a severe allergy should have the appropriate medication handy at all times. Ask your doctor if there are any medications that you should have available in case of an emergency.

artificial respiration
– infant (under one year)

- If the baby is pale, blue and obviously not breathing, **get medical help immediately**.

- If there is no one around to help you or to call 911 for you, administer the following procedure for one minute and then call for emergency help yourself.

- If you are not sure if the baby is breathing, look, listen and feel for signs of breathing (watch the chest for rising and falling, listen with your ear to the baby's mouth, and feel for the baby's breath on your ear).

- If the baby is not breathing, check for the pulse. If the pulse is present, go to Step 1. If there is no pulse, *see CPR on page 28*.

Procedure

1. Supporting the head and neck, gently place the baby onto his back on a flat surface, like a floor or table. Stand or kneel at the baby's side.

2. Look in the baby's mouth for foreign objects. Being extremely careful, remove anything from the mouth that you can see. Do not blindly poke around in the baby's mouth, as you may push an obstruction further into the airway or lungs.

3. If there is vomit or liquid in the mouth, roll the baby on one side so that the fluid can clear.

4. If you suspect that the baby may be choking, *see Choking on page 32*.

5. If you do not suspect a neck or back injury, place one hand on the baby's forehead and the fingers of your other hand under the chin. With one motion, lift the chin and gently press the forehead. This will clear the tongue from the back of the throat. The chin should not be up in the air nor down on the chest. You can roll a small towel and put it under the baby's neck. This will place the baby's head in the right position. Be careful not to press on the soft area under the chin or close the infant's mouth completely (keep your thumb in the infant's mouth if necessary, to keep the lips apart).

6. If you have any reason to believe that there might be a neck or back injury, open the airway by gently moving the baby's jaw forward. Do not tilt or move the baby's head.

7. Cover the baby's mouth and nose with your mouth, and make an airtight seal. Give two slow, gentle breaths, each about a second or a second-and-a-half in duration. Do not use more than the air in your cheeks, as more force may cause damage to a baby's lungs. Remove your mouth between breaths and wait for the baby's chest to fall before giving the next breath. *(See diagram A at right.)*

continued on next page

8. If you realize that the air isn't going in (if your breath feels blocked or if the baby's chest does not rise and fall), it is likely that the airway is blocked or your seal around the mouth and nose was not tight enough. Try to reopen the airway, repeating steps 1 to 7, or tighten your seal and try again. Give two more breaths, and if the air is still blocked, treat for choking. *See Choking, page 32.*

9. While continuing to hold the baby's head with one hand, check the pulse by pressing gently with the fingertips of your other hand on the inside of the upper arm between the elbow and shoulder. Do not use your thumb. Take up to 10 seconds to find a pulse. If you are feeling panicky, it is easy to miss.

10. If there is no pulse, *see CPR on page 28.*

11. If there is a pulse, give the infant another breath every three seconds, using slow, gentle breaths of between one and one-and-a-half seconds in duration, as described above, waiting for the chest to fall before giving the next breath. Check the pulse and look, listen and feel for breathing after the first minute of artificial respiration. Recheck every few minutes.

12. Continue giving breaths and checking pulse until the baby breathes on his own or professional help arrives.

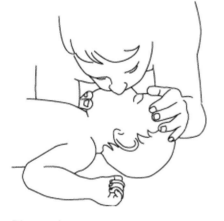

Diagram A

> **Note:** All parents are encouraged to take a CPR course from an accredited organization.

artificial respiration
– child (one year or older)

- If the child is pale, blue and obviously not breathing, **get medical help immediately.**

- If there is no one around to help you or to call 911 for you, administer the procedure described below for one minute and then call for emergency help yourself.

- If you are not sure if the child is breathing, look, listen and feel for signs of breathing (watch the chest for rising and falling, listen with your ear to the child's mouth, and feel for the child's breath on your ear).

- If the child is not breathing, check for pulse. If the pulse is present, go to Step 1 of the procedure. If there is no pulse, *see CPR on page 30.*

Procedure

1. Supporting the head and neck, gently place the child on his back on a flat surface, like a floor or table. Stand or kneel at the child's side.

2. Look in the child's mouth for foreign objects. Being extremely careful, remove anything from the mouth that you can see. Do not blindly poke around in the child's mouth, as you may push an obstruction further into the airway or lungs.

3. If there is vomit or liquid in the mouth, roll the child on one side so that the fluid can clear.

4. If you suspect that the child may be choking, *see Choking on page 34.*

5. If you do not suspect a neck or back injury, place one hand on the child's forehead and the fingers of your other hand under the chin. With one motion, lift the chin and gently press the forehead. This will clear the tongue from the back of the throat. The chin should not be up in the air nor down on the chest. You can roll a small towel and put it under the child's neck. This will place the child's head in the right position. Be careful not to press on the soft area under the chin or close the child's mouth completely (keep your thumb in the child's mouth, if necessary, to keep the lips apart).

6. If you have any reason to believe that there might be a neck or back injury, open the airway by gently moving the child's jaw forward. Do not tilt or move the head.

7. Pinch the child's nose closed with your thumb and fore-finger and place your open mouth tightly around the mouth forming a seal. Give two slow, gentle breaths, each about a second or a second-and-a-half in duration. Remove your mouth between breaths, and wait for the chest to fall before giving the next breath. *(See diagram A at right.)*

continued on next page

8. If you suspect that the air is not going in, (if your breath feels blocked, or if the child's chest does not rise and fall), it is likely that the airway is blocked or your seal around the mouth was not tight enough. Try to reopen the airway, repeating steps 1 to 7, or tighten your seal and try again. Give two more breaths, and if the air is still blocked, treat for choking. *See Choking, page 34.*

9. While continuing to hold the child's head with one hand, check the pulse by placing the fingertips of your other hand (but not your thumb) on the large artery on the side of the neck. Take five to ten seconds to find it – don't rush.

10. If there is no pulse, *see CPR on page 30.*

11. If there is a pulse, give the child a new breath every four seconds. Remove your mouth between breaths and wait for the chest to fall before giving the next breath. Check the pulse and look, listen and feel for breathing after the first minute of artificial respiration. Recheck every few minutes.

12. Continue giving breaths and checking the pulse until the child breathes on his own or professional help arrives.

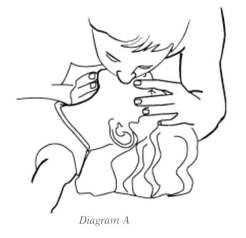

Diagram A

Note: All parents are encouraged to take a CPR course from an accredited organization.

bites and stings

insect stings & bites

- A severely allergic child should wear medical identification to warn of his condition, and carry a "sting kit" if prescribed by your doctor. If a severely allergic child has been bitten or stung, **get emergency medical help immediately** and *see Anaphylactic Shock on page 15.*

- You should be concerned if the insect sting or bite becomes infected and causes an allergic reaction, or if you suspect that the bite or sting was caused by a poisonous insect.

Procedure

1. **Get emergency medical attention immediately** if child has been bitten or stung by a *poisonous spider* or a *scorpion*.

2. Most other bites (from bedbugs, fleas, gnats and mosquitoes) should be washed with soap and water, and treated with cold compresses or calamine lotion to relieve minor swelling and itching.

3. For stings (wasps, bees, etc.), **get medical attention immediately** if the child has an allergic reaction (signs include hives-like rash, swollen hands, swollen eyelids, wheezing or difficulty breathing), or if there is severe swelling at the site of the sting. Severe allergic reactions will usually occur within an hour of the sting. Watch closely for any change in breathing. If the child has difficulty breathing, *see Anaphylactic Shock on page 15.*

> **Note:** If your child has a history of severe allergies to insect stings, you should discuss with your doctor desensitizing the child with a series of shots.

4. How to remove a stinger: A **bee** stinger has a venom sac attached. To remove the venom sac, scrape away the sac with your fingernail, the edge of a credit card or a blunt knife (don't squeeze with tweezers, as this will force the venom into the wound). Remove the rest of the stinger with tweezers. **Wasps, hornets and yellow jackets** do not have venom sacs. Remove stinger with tweezers.

5. After removing the stinger, apply an ice pack to the sting site to slow the spread of venom and ease the pain of the sting.

6. Watch closely for any signs of allergic reaction, especially if this is your child's first sting.

tick bites

- Ticks can carry disease (for example, the germ that causes Lyme disease), and they should be carefully and completely removed.

Procedure

1. Clean the area thoroughly with a cotton ball soaked with alcohol.

2. Grab the tick with tweezers, as close to the skin as possible, and slowly pull straight out, being careful not to twist or squeeze the tick (as it could break off and part of the tick could remain under the skin).

3. Save the tick if Lyme disease is prevalent in your area, and take it to your doctor to have it analyzed. (*Lyme disease is rare.*)

4. See your doctor if any part of the tick remains embedded or if, over the following days or months, the child develops any of the following symptoms – including muscle and joint pains and stiffness, swollen eyes, spots on hands and feet, dizziness, fatigue, chills and fever.

5. Clean the bite area again with antiseptic, rubbing alcohol or soap and water.

animal bites

- If the bite has penetrated the skin or there is severe bleeding, or if any signs of infection develop, **get medical attention immediately**.

- Call Animal Control or the police, who can check the animal for rabies.

Procedure

1. Control the bleeding by applying pressure on the wound with sterile gauze or a clean cloth. If necessary, *see Bleeding on page 22.*

2. Apply a sterile bandage and call your doctor immediately to find out about the possibility of rabies. If the bite is due to a bat, skunk, a fox or an unprovoked cat or dog, there is a possibility that the animal has rabies. A series of rabies vaccinations will be available if indicated.

3. Observe whether the child is in shock (symptoms include pale or blue lips and fingernails; clammy skin; weakness; deep and irregular or weak, shallow breathing). If symptoms of shock are present, *see Shock on page 45.*

bleeding

major bleeding

- **Get medical attention immediately.**

- Wash your hands and if possible put on sterile latex gloves.

Procedure

1. Speak calmly and reassuringly to the child.

2. Apply pressure to the wound for two minutes with sterile gauze or a clean cloth. Do not apply pressure to breaks, fractures or wounds containing embedded objects.

3. While applying pressure, elevate the site of the wound above the level of the heart if possible.

4. If possible, hold the wound under cold running water and assess the severity of the cut.

5. If only a small vein has been cut, bleeding will stop after two or three minutes of pressure.

6. If an artery has been cut, blood will spurt. Apply constant pressure for at least 10 minutes and elevate the wound to stop a bleeding artery. Do not release pressure to check on the wound, and be sure to keep it elevated.

7. Instead of removing gauze or cloth (which may dislodge the clot that has started to form and allow bleeding to begin again), place a second piece of gauze on top of the first, without removing pressure. Wrap tape around the bandage to keep pressure on the wound. Do not wrap it too tightly. Keep the bandage on for 20 minutes, then check the wound site to see if bleeding has subsided, and seek medical attention.

8. Observe whether child is in shock (symptoms include pale or blue lips and fingernails; clammy skin; weakness; deep and irregular or weak, shallow breathing). If symptoms of shock are present, *see Shock on page 45.*

minor bleeding

Procedure

1. Be calm and reassure the child that he is going to be fine. (Even a small cut is frightening to a child.)

2. Hold the cut under cold running water for a few minutes.

3. Even if the bleeding has stopped, apply an adhesive bandage to reassure the child that he is all better.

4. Keep the cut clean (depending on the type and location of the cut, your doctor may advise cleaning with hydrogen peroxide and using an antibiotic ointment daily to avoid infection).

broken or fractured bones

- Signs of broken or fractured bones are swelling, pain and limited movement and tenderness to the touch at the site of break or fracture.

- **Get medical attention immediately.**

- Do not try to straighten injured bones.

Procedure

1. If there is bleeding caused by a bone protruding through the skin, do not apply direct pressure to the site of the wound. Instead, control the bleeding by applying indirect pressure.

   Arm injury: Control bleeding by squeezing the upper arm, with your fingers on the inner arm between the two muscles. Cover the wound with a sterile dressing. Do not attempt to clean the wound.

   Leg injury: Control bleeding by applying firm pressure to the bone at the inner groin area at the crease of the leg. Cover the wound with a sterile dressing. Do not attempt to clean the wound.

2. **Do not move the child if there is a possibility of neck or back injury.**

3. Keep the child as still as possible until help arrives. Or, if you must take the child to the hospital or doctor's office, do not do so before immobilizing the break or fracture in the position found, using a sling or splint.

   Sling: If the collarbone or shoulder is broken, make sling to support the weight of the arm, with the hand positioned higher than the elbow.

   Splint (arm): You can make a splint out of a magazine, board or anything that will keep the arm in the position found. Pad the splint with cloth against the skin and bind it to the arm (not at the location of the injury), being careful not to tie it too tightly. Support the splint with a sling as described above.

   Splint (finger): Tape the injured finger to the next finger to hold it in place, or make a splint from a popsicle stick or emery board.

continued on next page

Splint (leg): Make a splint for the leg, padding and binding it to the leg as described above, out of a board or anything that will keep the injured leg from bending.

4. Observe whether the child is in shock (symptoms include pale or blue lips and fingernails; clammy skin; weakness; deep and irregular or weak, shallow breathing). If symptoms of shock are present, *see Shock on page 45.*

burns

first, second & third-degree

- The sooner you treat a burn, the better chance you have of reducing the damage to the skin.

- Speak to and act reassuringly with the child.

- For a minor burn inside the mouth, give the child an ice cube to suck on.

- **Get medical help immediately if:**
  - the burn involves the eyes, face, hands, genitals or airway; or
  - any signs of infection develop (including increased pain, swelling, pus or swollen glands).

- If the face has been burned, sit or prop the child up and apply a cool compress.

- If the child's clothes are on fire, smother fire with a blanket, towel or your body.

- Immediately remove any burning or hot-water-soaked clothing from the child. Do not touch any other part of the body with the hot clothing for fear of causing further burning. Remove clothes using scissors if necessary. Never attempt to remove clothing that has adhered to the skin.

- Never put butter, grease or powder on a burn.

- Give child acetaminophen if necessary for pain.

Procedure

1. Immediately immerse the burned area in cool water for at least 20 minutes, or gently apply a cool, wet towel until pain subsides. (Do not use ice, as this may cause further damage to the skin.) Cooling the burned skin arrests the burning process, which can go on under the surface if the upper layer is still hot.

2. Assess the burn, using the following symptoms as your guide, and proceed with the appropriate treatment:

first- and second-degree burns

- **Red or discolored skin, or blisters and red, swollen and peeling skin:**

1. Gently blot dry with a clean cloth.

2. If the burned area is only red (first-degree), leave it in cool water for up to 30 minutes, and then leave it uncovered, watching for change.

3. If there is blistering (second-degree), cover loosely with a dry, sterile, non-adhesive dressing or a clean, dry cloth, handkerchief or sheet. **Get medical help immediately**. Do not break blisters, as they protect the burned skin underneath.

third-degree burns

- **White or charred skin:**

1. **Get emergency medical help immediately.**

2. Cover loosely with sterile gauze or clean, dry cloth, handkerchief or sheet.

3. Check that the child is breathing and that there is a pulse. If not, *see Artificial Respiration on page 16 or CPR on page 28*.

4. Do not attempt to remove clothing that has adhered to the skin.

5. Do not remove tissue from the burn or break blisters.

6. Do not give the child anything to drink.

7. Elevate burned area higher than the heart (as this may help alleviate pain).

8. Check the child for signs of shock. *See Shock, page 45.*

chemical burns

- **Get medical help immediately.**

- Try to locate and identify the chemical causing the burn.

- If a chemical has been inhaled, swallowed or splashed into the eyes, call a poison control center or **emergency medical help immediately.**

- If a chemical has splashed in the child's eyes, flush eyes for 20 minutes with a steady stream of cool water from a pitcher. *See Eye Injuries, page 40.*

- Do not apply ointments unless advised to do so by your doctor or a poison control center.

- Try not to become contaminated yourself by the chemical.

- If signs of allergic reaction appear (rash, bright red lips and skin, dizziness, pain, difficulty breathing, headache), **get medical attention immediately.**

Procedure

1. Remove all contaminated clothing, being careful not to spread the irritant to other areas of the skin. Use scissors to cut away clothes if necessary, or leave clothing on if it cannot be removed safely.

2. Put burned area under cool running water for 20 minutes.

3. Wash area with soap and water, but do not scrub as this may cause chemical to be absorbed into the skin.

4. Apply cool compresses for pain relief.

5. Cover loosely with sterile dressing.

Note: If your clothes are ever set on fire: STOP, DROP to the ground and ROLL over and over until flames are out.

CPR (cardiopulmonary resuscitation)
– infant (under one year)

- If the baby is not breathing and has no pulse, **get emergency medical help immediately**.

- If there is no one around to help you or to call 911 for you, administer procedure below for one minute, and then call for emergency help yourself.

- If you have already administered artificial respiration, go immediately to Step 10.

> **Note:** All parents are encouraged to take a CPR course from an accredited organization.

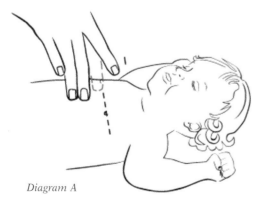

Diagram A

Procedure

1. Supporting the head and neck, gently place the baby onto his back on a flat surface, like a floor or table. Stand or kneel at the baby's side.

2. Look in the baby's mouth for foreign objects. Being extremely careful, remove anything from the mouth that you can see. Do not blindly poke around in the baby's mouth, as you may push an obstruction further into the airway or lungs.

3. If there is vomit or liquid in the mouth, roll the baby on one side so that the fluid can clear.

4. If you suspect that the baby may be choking, *see Choking on page 32.*

5. If you do not suspect a neck or back injury, place one hand on the baby's forehead and the fingers of your other hand under the chin. With one motion, lift the chin and gently press the forehead. This will clear the tongue from the back of the throat. The chin should not be up in the air nor down on the chest. You can roll a small towel and put it under the baby's neck. This will place the baby's head in the right position. Be careful not to press on the soft area under the chin or close the infant's mouth completely (keep your thumb in the mouth, if necessary, to keep the infant's lips apart).

6. If you have any reason to believe that there might be a neck or back injury, open the airway by gently moving the baby's jaw forward. Do not tilt or move the head.

continued on next page

7. Cover the baby's mouth and nose with your mouth. Give two slow, gentle breaths, each about a second or a second-and-a-half in duration. Do not use more than the air in your cheeks, as forcing too much air may cause damage to the baby's lungs. Remove your mouth between breaths and wait for the chest to fall before giving the next breath.

8. If you realize that the air isn't going in (if your breath feels blocked or if the chest does not rise and fall), it is likely that the airway is blocked or your seal around the mouth and nose was not tight enough. Try to reopen the airway, repeating steps 1 to 7, or tighten your seal and try again. Give two more breaths, and if the air is still blocked, treat for choking. *See Choking, page 32.*

9. While continuing to hold the head with one hand, check the baby's pulse by pressing gently with the fingertips of your other hand on the inside of the child's upper arm between the elbow and shoulder. Do not use your thumb. Take up to 10 seconds to find a pulse. If you are feeling panicked, it is easy to miss.

10. If you can't find a pulse, place two or three fingers midway between the infant's nipples, and one-finger width below an imaginary line that would join them. Do not push down on the lower tip of the breastbone. If you feel the tip, reposition your fingers further up the breastbone, closer to the imaginary line. *(See diagram A on page 28 at left).*
For a newborn, it may be easier if you encircle the baby's chest with your hands, just below the armpits, and compress the breastbone with your thumbs.

11. Make five short, downward compressions on the child's chest, one-half to one inch deep, taking about a half a second for each. Thrust down, not from side to side. *Do not remove your fingertips between compressions.*

12. Keeping your fingertips in place, stop and give the infant a slow, gentle breath (one to one-and-a-half seconds in duration).

13. Continue giving five compressions and one breath. To be sure that you are doing this at the right rate, count out loud –"One and two and three and four and five…" – and then breathe.

14. Check the pulse and then look, listen and feel for breathing after the first minute of artificial respiration. Recheck every few minutes.

15. Once the pulse is restored, stop compressions.

16. Keep giving the child breaths until he breathes on his own or until professional help arrives.

CPR (cardiopulmonary resuscitation)
– child (one year or older)

- If the child is not breathing and has no pulse, **get emergency medical help immediately.**

- If there is no one around to help you or to call 911 for you, administer procedure below for one minute and then call for emergency help yourself.

- If you have already administered artificial respiration, go immediately to Step 10.

> **Note:** All parents are encouraged to take a CPR course from an accredited organization.

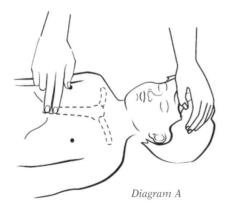

Diagram A

Procedure

1. Supporting the head and neck, gently place the child onto his back on a flat surface, like a floor or table. Stand or kneel at his side.

2. Look in the child's mouth for foreign objects. Being extremely careful, remove anything from the mouth that you can see. Do not blindly poke around in the child's mouth, as you may push an obstruction further into the airway or lungs.

3. If there is vomit or liquid in the mouth, roll the child on one side so that the fluid can clear.

4. If you suspect that the child may be choking, *see Choking on page 34.*

5. If you do not suspect a neck or back injury, place one hand on the child's forehead and the fingers of your other hand under the chin. With one motion, lift the chin and gently press the forehead. This will clear the tongue from the back of the throat. The chin should not be up in the air nor down on the chest. You can roll a small towel and put it under the child's neck. This will place the child's head in the right position. Be careful not to press on the soft area under the chin or close the child's mouth completely (keep your thumb in the mouth, if necessary, to keep the lips apart).

6. If you have any reason to believe that there might be a neck or back injury, open the airway by gently moving the child's jaw forward. Do not tilt or move his head.

7. Pinch the child's nose closed with your thumb and forefinger and place your open mouth tightly around the mouth, forming a seal. Give two slow, gentle breaths, each about one second or a second-and-a-half in duration. Remove your mouth between breaths, and wait for the chest to fall before giving the next breath.

continued on next page

8. If you realize that the air isn't going in (if your breath feels blocked, or if the child's chest does not rise and fall), it is likely that the airway is blocked or your seal around his mouth was not tight enough. Try to reopen the airway, repeating steps 1 to 7, or tighten your seal and try again. Give two more breaths, and if the air is still blocked, treat for choking. *See Choking on page 34.*

9. While continuing to hold the child's head with one hand, check the pulse by placing the fingertips of your other hand (but not your thumb) on the large artery on the side of the neck. Take five to ten seconds to find it – don't rush.

10. If you can't find a pulse, place two or three fingers midway between the child's nipples, and one-finger width below an imaginary line that would join them. *(See diagram A on page 30 at left).*

11. Lift your fingers off the breastbone and place the heel of the same hand just above the point where the top of your index finger was. *(See diagram B on this page.)*

12. Keeping the child's head in the same position with your hand on the forehead, make **five** short, downward compressions on the chest, one to one-and-a-half inches deep, taking about three-fourths of a second for each. Thrust straight down, not from side to side. *Do not remove your hand between compressions.*

13. Stop *every five compressions*, remove your hand from the child's chest and lift the chin. Pinch the nose closed with the hand that was on the child's forehead and give a slow, gentle breath (one to one-and-a-half seconds in duration). Now put the heel of your hand back on the child's chest in the *exact* position as before.

Diagram B of downward compressions

14. Continue the process of five compressions and one breath. To be sure that you are doing this at the right rate, count out loud – "One and two and three and four and five…" – and then breathe.

15. Check the pulse and then look, listen and feel for breathing after the first minute of artificial respiration. Recheck every few minutes.

16. Once the pulse is restored, stop compressions.

17. Keep giving the child breaths until he breathes on his own or until professional help arrives.

choking
– infant (under one year)

- If an infant cannot cough, cry or take in any air (gasping, turning blue or fainting from choking), **get emergency medical help immediately.**

- If there is no one around to help you or to call 911 for you, administer the procedures described below for one minute and then call for emergency help yourself.

- If the infant **can** cough, cry and breathe, this is a sign that his reflexes are working to free the obstruction for him. Do not interfere, as following any of the intervention procedures below may force the piece further into his airway or lungs. Watch the infant closely for signs that he can no longer attempt to free the obstruction on his own, and be sure to calm and reassure the baby, as panic may make his effort more difficult.

- If you can see the obstruction, remove it carefully with your finger. Do not sweep blindly for objects that you can't see, as this may cause the piece to go further into his airway or lungs.

- If the infant can't free the obstruction on his own, use the following procedure:

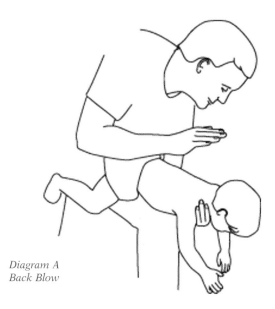

Diagram A
Back Blow

Note: If vomiting should occur at any point, immediately turn the infant on his side, clear the mouth with your finger and resume rescue procedure.

★ After any choking episode, be sure to have your doctor examine the baby.

★ All parents are encouraged to take a CPR course from an accredited organization.

Procedure

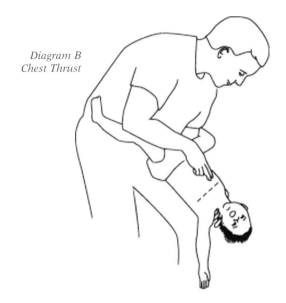

*Diagram B
Chest Thrust*

1. Position the infant, **face down**, along the length of your forearm, supporting the chin in your hand. Hold your arm at an angle, so the head is lower than the rest of the body.

2. With your thigh bent forward under your forearm for support, use the heel of your other hand to give the infant four quick back blows between the shoulder blades. *(See diagram A at left.)*

3. If the obstruction does not clear or if the baby does not begin to cough or cry, flip him over so that he is **face up** along your forearm. Support the head with your hand and keep the head lower than the rest of the body. Again, rest your arm on your thigh for support.

4. Place two or three fingers of your other hand midway between the infant's nipples, and one-finger width below an imaginary line that would join them. Make four quick thrusts downward on the infant's chest, one-half to one inch deep. Thrust down, not from side to side. Allow the breastbone to return to normal position before giving the next thrust. Do not remove your fingers between thrusts. *(See diagram B above.)*

5. If the baby is still not breathing or has not dislodged the obstruction, depress the baby's tongue with your thumb, and with the tongue and jaw between thumb and fore-finger, lift the jaw up and open to inspect the back of the baby's throat. By pulling the tongue away from the throat, you may relieve the obstruction. If you can see the obstruction, sweep it out with your finger, but again be careful not to push it further back into the throat. *(See diagram C.)*

6. If the baby is still not breathing, cover the baby's mouth *and nose* with your mouth. Give two slow, gentle breaths, each about a second or a second-and-a-half in duration. Do not use more than the air in your cheeks, as forcing more air may cause damage to the baby's lungs. If you see the baby's chest rise and fall, you know the air-way is clear. Continue giving gentle breaths until the baby is breathing on his own.

7. If the airway is not clear, repeat back blows, chest thrusts, mouth-check and breaths until professional help arrives, or until baby is breathing on his own and the obstruction is cleared.

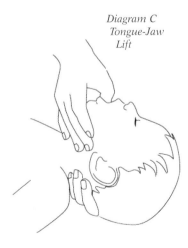

*Diagram C
Tongue-Jaw
Lift*

choking
– conscious child (one year or older)

- If a child cannot cough, cry or take in any air (gasping, turning blue, or fainting from choking), **get emergency medical help immediately.**

- If there is no one around to help you or to call 911 for you, administer the procedure described below for one minute and then call for emergency help yourself.

- If the child **can** cough, cry and breathe, this is a sign that his reflexes are working to free the obstruction for him. Do not interfere, as following any of the intervention procedures on this page may force the obstruction further into his airway or lungs. Watch the child closely for signs that he can no longer attempt to free the obstruction on his own, and be sure to calm and reassure the child, as panic may make his effort more difficult.

- If you can see the obstruction, remove it carefully with your finger. Do not sweep blindly for objects that you can't see, as this may cause the piece to go further into the child's airway or lungs.

- If the child can't free the obstruction on his own, place him in a sitting or standing position.

> **Note:** If vomiting should occur at any point, clear the child's mouth with your finger and resume rescue procedures.
>
> ★ After any choking episode, be sure to have your doctor examine the child.
>
> ★ All parents are encouraged to take a CPR course from an accredited organization.

Procedure

1. Stand or kneel behind the child and wrap your arms around his waist.

2. Form a fist with one hand and place the thumb of your fist against the child's abdomen, above the navel and well below the breastbone. Do not put your fist on the child's breastbone or ribs, as this may cause injury.
(See diagram A below.)

3. Hold onto your fist with your other hand and thrust quickly inward and upward with a jerking "J" motion. Be careful to thrust straight up, not to either side. Repeat *six to ten times* if necessary. Between each thrust, check to see if the object has been expelled, or if the child begins to cough or breathe.

4. If the object does not dislodge, or if the child does not begin to cough, check to make sure the child is still conscious. Readjust your hands if you determine that they are not in exactly the right position. Repeat the thrusts until the object is dislodged or until professional help arrives.

Diagram A

choking
– unconscious child (one year or older)

- If a child is unconscious, and you suspect he is choking (if he is not breathing, turning blue), **get emergency medical help immediately**.

- If there is no one around to help you, or to call 911 for you, administer the following procedure for one minute and then call for emergency help yourself.

- If you can see the obstruction, remove it carefully with your finger. Do not sweep blindly for objects that you can't see, as this may cause the piece to go further into the child's airway or lungs.

Procedure

1. Place the child on his back on a flat surface, like a floor or table.

2. Kneel or stand at his side or at his feet. If you straddle the child, your thrusts may be too forceful and you may injure him.

3. Place the heel of your hand on the child's abdomen, above the navel and well below the breastbone with your fingers facing the chin. Do not put your hand on the breastbone or ribs, as this may cause injury. *(See diagram A below.)*

4. Place your other hand on top of the first hand, and give *six to ten* quick downward and forward thrusts to the abdomen. Adjust your thrusts to the size of the child, being more gentle for a smaller child.

5. If the obstruction does not come out of the child's mouth, or if he does not begin to cough or breathe, depress the tongue with your thumb, and with the tongue and jaw between your thumb and forefinger, lift the jaw up and open to inspect the back of the child's throat. By pulling the tongue away from the throat, you may relieve the obstruction. If you can see the obstruction, sweep it out with your finger, but again be careful not to push it further back into the throat.

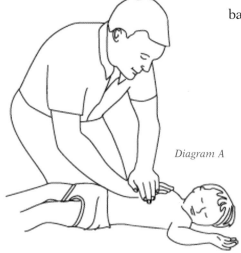

Diagram A

continued on next page

6. If the child is still not breathing, pinch the child's nose closed with your thumb and forefinger and place your open mouth tightly around his mouth forming a seal. Give two slow, gentle breaths, each about a second or a second-and-a-half in duration. If the child's chest rises, the airway is clear. Continue giving breaths until the child begins to breathe on his own.

7. If the airway is not clear, repeat chest thrusts, mouth-check and breaths until professional help arrives, or until child is breathing on his own and the obstruction is cleared.

Note: If vomiting should occur at any point, immediately turn the child on his side, clear the mouth with your finger and resume rescue procedures.

★ After any choking episode, be sure to have your doctor examine the child.

★ All parents are encouraged to take a CPR course from an accredited organization.

convulsions and seizures

- Stay as calm as possible.

- During a convulsion, a child may experience jerky, uncontrollable movements or muscle spasms, writhe on the ground, bite his tongue, froth at the mouth, temporarily lose consciousness, roll his eyes.

- Don't give the child anything to eat or drink during or immediately following the convulsion. Don't put anything in the child's mouth (including your fingers).

- Most convulsions in babies are caused by fever. To prevent further convulsions due to fever, give an acetaminophen suppository (giving it by mouth may cause the child to choke).

- Do not try to restrain the child from shaking.

- **Get medical attention** after all convulsions and seizures.

Procedure

1. Ensure that the child cannot hurt himself.

2. Gently place him on the floor, on his side. Turn his head to one side. This will allow secretions to leave the mouth and the tongue to come forward.

3. Make sure that there is no constraining clothing around the child's neck that could become tighter with the jerking and shaking movements of a convulsion.

4. Clear the area around the convulsing child of anything that could harm him should he bump into it.

5. Watch the child closely to make sure he is breathing. If he is not breathing, *See Artificial Respiration, page 16.*

6. Call for **medical emergency attention** if the convulsion lasts more than five minutes.

> **Note:** After a convulsion or seizure, check the child for injuries and call your doctor.

electric shock

- Do not try to remove the child from an electric current with your bare hands.

- **Get medical help immediately** following an electric shock.

Procedure

1. Switch off all electrical power sources. If there is a wall socket, turn it off or unplug cord.

2. If it is not possible to quickly turn off the power source, immediately remove child from current with a non-metallic object, like a broom, cushion, chair or board.

3. Check that the child is breathing and that he has a pulse. If necessary, begin artificial respiration or CPR until child revives or medical help arrives. *See Artificial Respiration, page 16 or CPR on page 28.*

> **Note:** Electrical currents can cause irregular heartbeats or burns to tissue. Get medical attention after an electric shock to find out if there are any injuries which you cannot see.

eye injuries

- When a foreign object gets stuck in a child's eye, symptoms can include a burning sensation, excessive tearing, itching, overall redness, sensitivity to light and increased prominence of the blood vessels in the whites of the eye.

- Do not try to remove a foreign object in the eye with tweezers or cotton balls.

- Foreign bodies can scratch the surface of the eye and should therefore be removed as soon as possible to prevent further damage. **Get medical help immediately** if the object is on the iris or pupil, or seems to be embedded in the eye.

- Always wash your hands thoroughly before administering any first aid to the eyes.

- To keep a baby from rubbing the eyes, wrap him with his arms secured inside a towel, blanket or sheet. Then begin treatment.

Procedure

1. Gently pull down the upper eyelid over the lower eyelid and allow a flow of tears to flush the eye.

2. If this does not work, flush the child's eyes. It is best to have two people – someone to hold the child and someone to flush the eye. Lay the child down on the side of the affected eye, with a towel placed under the head. Gently pull down the child's lower eyelid and encourage child to open his eyes very wide as you irrigate them with a gentle, steady stream of lukewarm water from a clean pitcher. Allow the water to run across the eye and onto the towel.

3. If the child has splashed a chemical irritant into the eye, continue flushing for at least 15 minutes.

4. Do not attempt to remove a foreign body from the surface of the eyeball. This should be done by a doctor. Never use a dry tissue, cotton swab or tweezers near the eye.

5. If medical treatment is not available and the foreign body is extremely irritating, try to locate it by gently pulling down the child's lower eyelid and asking the child to look up. If the foreign object is still not visible, lift the upper eyelid and have the child look down.

6. Once you locate the irritant, try to remove it with a wet corner of a clean piece of cloth (not a tissue, as this may break apart and stay in the child's eye).

7. Following treatment, call for medical advice. Some corrosives may irritate the cornea and promote infection. Preventative antibiotic ointment may be needed. Pain from a scratch or irritant may last for 24 hours. If the eye still hurts, the foreign body may not have been completely removed or the eyeball has been scratched and needs medical attention.

head injuries

- Always observe your child carefully after any incident which results in a head injury. How the child reacts or behaves **after** the injury may indicate whether or not he has a concussion or other brain injury.

bumps and "goose eggs"

- A bump, a goose egg or a swelling on the scalp is caused by broken blood vessels under the skin and are seldom cause for concern of underlying brain injury.

- If the child is alert, conscious and acting as he was before the injury, proceed to Step 1 of procedure.

Procedure

1. Apply ice packs and pressure to the goose egg for 20 minutes.

2. Watch the child closely for changes in behavior (a change in breathing, color of skin becoming pale or blue, change in breathing pattern, loss of balance and coordination, twitches on one side of the body, persistent vomiting, crossed or rolling eyes).

3. Call your doctor with any observations that concern you.

scalp bleeds

- The scalp is likely to bleed profusely if cut. As explained above, this is seldom cause for concern of brain injury unless it is caused by a puncture.

Procedure

1. Apply pressure to the site of the cut using sterile gauze or a clean cloth for two minutes. *See Bleeding, page 22.*

2. Assess the cut. If the cause is a puncture, **get medical help immediately**, as infection to the brain may occur from such an injury.

3. Watch the child closely for changes in behavior (a change in breathing, color of skin becoming pale or blue, change in breathing pattern, loss of balance and coordination, twitches on one side of the body, persistent vomiting, crossed or rolling eyes).

4. Call your doctor with any observations that concern you.

Concussions on next page.

concussion/bleeding in the brain (brain injury)

- **Symptoms of brain injury include:** disorientation; difficulty waking up or being awakened; confusion; unusual breathing pattern while sleeping (irregular, shallow breaths); crossed or rolling eyes or unequal pupils; increased paleness; persistent vomiting; convulsions; loss of balance while sitting, crawling or walking; loss of coordination in hand movements; blood or watery fluid oozing from the ear.

- If a child has any of these symptoms in the 24 hours following a blow to the head, there may be an injury to the brain. **Get medical attention immediately.**

- Call your doctor for advice on how long to observe your child and what to observe. This will depend on the age of your child and the type of injury.

nose injuries

- A child's nose acts as shock absorber for blows to the face and often prevents serious damage to the head. After most injuries, the nose returns to normal without being deformed.

- If the nose is pushed to the side and becomes crooked, or if air flow seems to be blocked or impaired, **get medical attention**.

Procedure

1. Put an ice pack gently on the child's nose, lightly pressing on the swollen area on each side of the nose just below the corners of the eyes. The sooner after an injury that ice is applied on the nose, the less the nose will swell.

2. Ice for at least 20 minutes. The longer the ice pack is applied, the less the swelling will be.

nose bleeds

- Do not lean a child back, or lay him down, as blood may drip down his throat causing him to vomit or sneeze and release the clot.

- **Get medical attention** if a nosebleed persists after taking the following procedure:

Procedure

1. Have child sit on your lap and lean **forward** slightly.

2. You can twist a piece of wet cotton and insert it into the bleeding nostril so that it fills two-thirds of the opening. If you chose not to use a cotton packing, the recommended procedure in all nose bleed cases will be the following: pinch the soft part of nostrils together for at least 10 minutes without releasing. (Do not pinch the bony part because this will not be effective.) If your child needs a cotton packing to stop the bleeding, he should be examined by his doctor.

3. If the bleeding hasn't stopped, place a piece of wet cotton under the upper lip and apply pressure with two fingers under the lip, pointing in the direction of the nostrils, or over the upper lip just below the nostrils. This is where the major blood vessel supplying the nose is located.

4. Once the bleeding stops, if you have used a cotton packing, leave the cotton in the nose for a few hours, allowing the clot to form. Gently remove the cotton. If the cotton is difficult to remove, wet it slightly with water so as not to dislodge the clot and restart the nosebleed.

poisoning

- Try to identify and keep handy the source of poison.

- **Call your poison control center, hospital emergency room or 911 immediately.** Do not wait for symptoms to appear.

- Pay careful attention for any symptoms your child may have (such as coughing and vomiting).

- Do not induce vomiting unless instructed to do so by medical personnel or a poison control center. Inducing vomiting after ingesting some poisons may cause serious harm to your child.

- You may be advised by a poison control center to induce vomiting, or dilute the poison with water. Follow their directions closely.

- If the child has inhaled a poisonous substance, get the child to fresh air and **get medical help immediately.**

- If you are not sure if the child has been poisoned, but there are signs of possible poisoning (such as burns, stains or powders around child's mouth, or pills, poisonous plants or chemicals in the vicinity), **call a poison center immediately.**

- If the child is having any difficulty breathing, has a change in skin color, or begins to lose consciousness, **take him immediately to the emergency room.**

shock

- Whenever a child has been seriously injured, always treat for shock.

- The severity of shock depends on the duration and cause of the decrease in blood pressure, which is what sends the body into shock.

- If the cause of shock is minor (a minor burn, injury or emotional distress), blood pressure will return to normal within a half-hour.

- If the cause of shock is major (severe bleeding, burns, brain injury), **immediate medical help is needed.**

- **Get medical attention immediately** if any of the following symptoms are present: pale or blue lips and fingernails; clammy skin; weakness; deep and irregular or weak, shallow breathing.

- Make sure the child is warm but not overheated, and do not use hot water bottles or heating pads, etc.

- Do not give the child any food or water.

Procedure

1. Speak calmly and reassuringly to the child.

2. Lay the child down on his side and loosen any tight or constricting clothing.

3. **Do not move the child if there is a possibility of neck or back injury.**

4. If he has a head injury or if he is having trouble breathing, stabilize his head and elevate his head and shoulders, not just the head.

5. Cover child lightly with a blanket or coat to preserve body heat.

strains and sprains

Procedure

• **Get medical attention if:**

- you suspect a broken bone;

- pain is severe; or

- pain or swelling doesn't decrease after 24 hours.

1. Immediately after injury occurs, apply an ice pack to the injured area for at least 20 minutes. Reapply at regular intervals until swelling has subsided.

2. Compress the swollen area by wrapping the ice pack with an elastic bandage. Make the wrap snug but not constricting.

3. Elevate the limb on a pillow or support it with a sling to prevent it from moving or bearing any weight.

sunburn

- Get the child out of the sun immediately.

- If the skin is blistered, **get medical attention immediately.** *See Burns on page 26* for second-degree burn treatment.

- If eyelids are burned, **get medical attention.**

- If skin is only slightly red and child seems comfortable, no treatment is needed.

- If skin is extremely red and the child is uncomfortable, use the following procedure:

Procedure

1. Immerse burned skin in cool water or use cool wet compresses or towels for at least 15 minutes, 4 times a day.

2. Do not dry the skin. Let the water evaporate and cool the burn.

3. Apply a non-petroleum moisturizer, such as aloe, to the affected area(s) several times a day.

4. If child is in pain, give acetaminophen.

5. Make sure the child's clothes or bedsheets do not irritate painful skin.

Note: If you suspect that the child has sunstroke (signs include dizziness, sickness, sudden high fever, confusion), *see Sunstroke on page 48.*

---

sunstroke or heat stroke

- Sunstroke or heat stroke can be fatal if not treated immediately – the child's body temperature must be lowered quickly. **Get medical attention immediately.**

- Symptoms include dizziness, sickness, sudden high fever and confusion.

- Removing the child from the sun or source of heat will not cure the condition.

- Do not give the child any medication without the advice of a doctor.

- Observe whether child is in shock (symptoms include pale or blue lips, gums and fingernails; clammy, mottled skin; weakness; weak and shallow or deep, irregular breathing). If symptoms of shock are present, *see Shock on page 45.*

Procedure

1. Wrap child in cool wet towels, apply cool compresses to his body, or place him in bathtub with cool water and lightly sponge his entire body.

2. When child's temperature is reduced to near-normal, dry him off. Give him something to drink to replace lost fluids.

3. Watch the child closely and repeat the treatment if temperature rises again or symptoms reappear.

record of medical emergencies

Date   **Record here any medical emergencies and how they were treated**

continued on next page

record of medical emergencies

Date   **Record here any medical emergencies and how they were treated**

notes

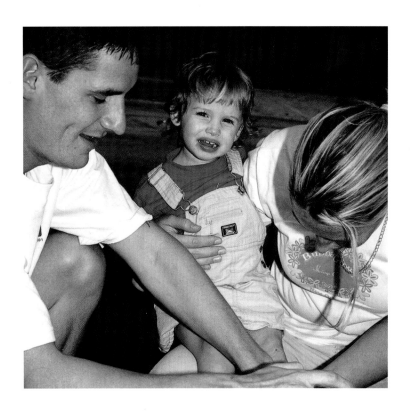

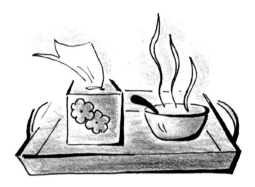

childhood illnesses

introduction

Information is your most important resource as a parent – quickly followed by your own intuition – when it comes to your children's health and safety. This is particularly true when your children are too young to explain their symptoms verbally.

In the following section of this book, the childhood illnesses are listed in alphabetical order, followed by symptoms, treatment suggestions and special information worth noting. All of this will help you to assess your child's condition as quickly as possible, and to know whether to begin treatment on your own or seek medical attention immediately.

NOTE: It is important to remember that this book will provide you with basic information only – always consult your doctor if you are concerned.

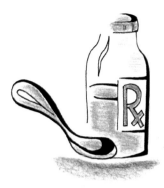

list of childhood illnesses

in alphabetical order

- Anemia
- Appendicitis
- Asthma
- Boils
- Bronchiolitis
- Bronchitis
- Cellulitis
- Chicken Pox
- Clogged tear duct
- Common cold
- Conjunctivitis
- Croup
- Diaper rash
- Diarrhea
- Diphtheria
- Ear infection

- Epiglottitis
- Fifth disease
- Flu
- German measles
- Hand, foot and mouth syndrome
- Head lice
- Herpangina
- Herpes simplex
- Hives
- Impetigo
- Infectious mononucleosis
- Lyme disease
- Measles
- Meningitis
- Mumps

- Pinworms
- Pneumonia
- RSV (respiratory synctial virus)
- Reye's syndrome
- Roseola
- Scabies
- Scarlet fever
- Sinusitis
- Strep throat
- Tetanus
- Thrush
- Tonsillitis
- Urinary tract infection
- Whooping cough

Illness	Symptoms	Treatment	Worth Noting
Anemia	Paleness, especially on earlobes, lips and under fingernails; irritability; tiredness; slow growth; diminished appetite.	Prescription of iron drops or tablets; iron-rich foods; iron-fortified cereals; organ meats; fish.	• Drink juice with meals. • Vitamin C enhances iron absorption from the food.
Appendicitis	Vomiting; fever; loss of appetite; increasingly severe lower abdominal pain beginning around the navel and then localizing to the right side; hurts when child walks or jumps; child winces when you press on painful site.	**Seek medical attention immediately.**	• It's important to diagnose early. • Many cases of appendicitis in children rupture before they are diagnosed and treated.
Asthma	Labored breathing; indrawing (when you can see outline of ribs every time child breathes in); pale features; fatigue that increases with exertion; wheezing; cough; difficulty exhaling.	**Seek medical attention.** Do not attempt to treat first attack at home. Subsequent attacks may be treated by doctor's prescribed home treatment.	• Asthma can be a chronic condition. • Well-treated asthmatic children can enjoy a normal life and may outgrow the condition. • Asthma is not diagnosed until repeated episodes have been noted. • Asthma attacks generally get less severe and less frequent as child gets older. • Learn about and avoid factors which cause childhood incidents of asthma.

Illness	Symptoms	Treatment	Worth Noting
Boils	Swellings on skin that are red, raised, tender and filled with pus – usually on buttocks.	Apply hot compresses or warm Epsom-salts solution 10 times daily. Frequently clean surrounding skin with soap and water. Continue until after boil has popped and drained. Doctor may incise and drain.	• Try to keep from picking or squeezing the boil, as scarring or spreading might result. • Do not let drainage from a boil come into contact with eyes. • If boils develop on face, see your doctor. • If boils occur regularly, see your child's doctor as a topical medicine can be prescribed to prevent recurrences.
Bronchiolitis (in children under six months of age)	Cough; wheezing; labored breathing; decreased appetite; low-grade fever; irritability; bluish skin; tiredness; nasal congestion.	**Seek medical attention** if you notice increasing tiredness or decreased appetite. **Bluish skin coloration needs urgent medical attention.**	• Bronchiolitis can be a serious illness. Your child may require hospitalization. • Guard against dehydration. • Do not give cough medicine to a child who is having trouble breathing.
Bronchitis (in children over six months of age)	Decreased appetite; low-grade fever; cold symptoms; labored breathing; rapid breathing; irritability; bluish skin; tiredness; paleness; hacking cough; weakness; nasal congestion; wheezing.	See your doctor; rest; acetaminophen for fever; cool-mist humidifier; small, frequent feedings; increased liquids; phenylephrine or oxymetalozine nose drops.	• If there is pain on the side of the chest, or blood in the discharge coughed up, **see your doctor immediately**. • Do not give oral decongestants.

Note: Many children with hacking cough, or repeated diagnosis of bronchitis &/or pneumonia are undiagnosed asthmatics. Check with your doctor.

Illness	Symptoms	Treatment	Worth Noting
Cellulitis	Low-grade fever; swellings on skin that are red, raised, tender; swollen and tender local lymph glands.	See your doctor for assessment and treatment.	• It's important to treat cellulitis aggressively to prevent spreading into joints and bones.
Chicken pox (Varicella)	Itchy rash on trunk that begins like insect bites and then rapidly forms into blisters and spreads over trunk, face and mouth; low-grade fever. There may be mild cold symptoms.	Calamine lotion without phenol or Benadryl, administered with a soft cloth; Aveeno-treated lukewarm baths; acetaminophen to treat the fever or pain. Cut fingernails to lessen scratching.	• If pocks become infected, lymph nodes become red and tender, or unexplained bruises or broken blood vessels appear under skin, call your doctor. • Chicken pox is contagious until all pocks form into scabs. • Check with your doctor to ask about a vaccine to prevent the Chicken Pox.
Clogged tear duct	Excessive tearing in eyes of a generally well infant; occurs in only one eye; either constant or recurrent.	Gently massage in an upward direction toward the nose just beneath the tiny "bump" in the nasal corner of each eye. Call your doctor for antibiotic eye drops or ointment if excessive tearing is accompanied by persistent yellow discharge.	• Most clogged tear ducts open themselves but may need probing by an eye doctor if they haven't opened by nine months.

Illness	Symptoms	Treatment	Worth Noting
Common cold	Dry cough; low-grade or no fever; sneezing; watery eyes; runny nose.	Plenty of liquids; vaporizer or humidifier; cessation of vigorous activities; nose drops or oral decongestants and nasal aspirator to relieve congestion; cough medicine if cough is severe. (Consult your doctor for appropriate dosage of all medications for your child's age.)	• Do not overuse cold or cough medications. • Use nose drops or nasal decongestants with caution. They can be associated with arrhythmia in young children. • Do not expose young infants to anyone with a cold.
Conjunctivitis	Yellow drainage from eyes; red, swollen eyelids; itching, watery eyes; sneezing; bloodshot eyes; burning sensation; sensitivity to light; eyes that are "glued" shut in the morning.	Strict hand washing and prompt treatment are required. Call your doctor. Wash eyes with cool water. Apply warm compresses pressed lightly on eyes to relieve discomfort.	• Treat both eyes, even if only one appears to be infected.
Croup	"Seal bark" cough resulting from inflammation and swelling of the vocal cords and windpipe. Hoarse voice.	Humidity from shower or vaporizer. Help child relax or go to sleep. Give lots of fluids. Take child outside.	• If child is happy and smiling and having no difficulty getting air in, croup is not serious. • Watch the little dent in child's neck just above the breastbone. If it caves in with each labored breath and child seems to be either extremely tired or panicky, **seek medical attention immediately.**

Illness	Symptoms	Treatment	Worth Noting
Diaper rash	Red, raised, often itchy rash over diaper area.	Air baby's bottom with diapers off. Change diapers frequently. Rinse bottom well; blot-dry gently with cotton towel or diaper. Apply an over-the-counter zinc-oxide cream as a barrier.	• A diaper rash that persists despite the treatment described earlier could be a yeast infection. See your doctor.
Diarrhea	Increased stool amount and liquidity; stool that is light brown, yellow or green in color and may contain partially digested food; may be associated with a raw red rash around the anus; abdominal pain; nausea; vomiting; low-grade fever.	Give clear fluids (or oral electrolyte solutions) frequently. If still nursing, continue breastfeeding. Have child rest. **Call your doctor immediately** if child has severe abdominal pain or if you suspect dehydration – signs include drowsiness, inability to retain liquids, persistent diarrhea, blood in stool, vomiting, high fever, or decreased urination accompanying diarrhea.	• Do not give child any medication unless advised to do so by your doctor. • Usually caused by gastrointestinal infections, colds, food intolerances or antibiotic treatment. • Guard carefully against dehydration, which can be a serious medical emergency (especially in babies), by giving plenty of fluids.
Diphtheria	Low-grade fever; slightly or largely swollen glands under the jaw; inflamed tonsils; white membrane covering tonsils; difficulty breathing and swallowing; pus in throat; cough.	**Seek medical attention;** give fluids, popsicles, bland diet.	• Very rare, especially in immunized countries. • If child is having trouble breathing, do not attempt to look in his throat. • You can prevent diphtheria by getting your children immunized. Check with your doctor and local health department for immunization and vaccination information.

Illness	Symptoms	Treatment	Worth Noting
Ear infection	Earache, crankiness, waking-up crying and ear drainage, especially during a cold.	Prop child upright. Give acetaminophen for pain. Notify your doctor and have child's ears examined – doctor may prescribe antibiotic.	• To relieve pain of middle-of-the-night earaches, give appropriate dosage of acetaminophen. Squirt a few drops of warm cooking oil or olive oil into sore ear and massage outer edge of ear canal to move the drips down toward eardrum to relieve pain. Encourage child to lie with sore ear up. • Be sure to have child's ears re-examined by your doctor once a course of antibiotics has been finished, and on a regular basis if infections recur.
Epiglottitis	Difficulty breathing and swallowing; high-grade fever (103°F or higher); panicky demeanor; choking behavior (leans forward, sticks out tongue, drools); low-pitched cough; indrawing (when you can see outline of ribs every time child breathes in).	**Medical emergency – rush child to hospital.**	• Usually – but not always – occurs in children older than two years. • You can prevent epiglottitis by getting your children immunized. Check with your doctor and local health department for immunization and vaccination information.
Fifth disease	Low-grade fever; bright red rash that looks like "slapped cheeks"; lace-like rash on trunk and extremities; sore joints; itching.	Check with your doctor.	• Treatment is for comfort only; not a serious affliction.

Illness	Symptoms	Treatment	Worth Noting
Flu (influenza)	Achiness; low-grade fever; runny nose; diarrhea; vomiting; cough; general look of unwellness; chills; flushing; headache; sore throat; pain in back and limbs.	See your doctor. Bed rest; plenty of fluids; ice chips; small, frequent feedings; acetaminophen; isolation. You may give oral electrolyte solutions if the child has vomiting &/or diarrhea.	• The flu is commonly misdiagnosed over the phone – it requires a doctor's exam. • Do not give aspirin. • Don't assume child is well if fever disappears for a day; it could very well return.
German measles (rubella, three-day measles)	Slightly decreased appetite; pinkish-red spotted rash on face which spreads rapidly to trunk and disappears by the third day; low-grade fever; swollen glands behind ears and back of neck; slight redness of throat and whites of eyes.	Bed rest; plenty of liquids; ice chips; small, frequent feedings; acetaminophen to relieve fever; oral electrolyte solutions; isolation (especially from pregnant women).	• You can prevent rubella by getting your children immunized. Check with your doctor and local health department for immunization and vaccination information. • If you are pregnant and your prenatal screening blood test shows that you are not protected against German measles, be sure to receive your vaccine right after delivery.
Hand, foot and mouth syndrome	Low-grade fever; tiny, blister-like sores in the mouth, palms of hands and soles of feet; sore throat.	Plenty of liquids; soft foods; acetaminophen.	• Not serious; more of a nuisance than a medical concern. • Contagious.

Illness	Symptoms	Treatment	Worth Noting
Head lice	Lice can rarely be seen except with a magnifying glass; however, their egg sacs (which are whitish nits) attach to base of hair strand; can be distinguished from dandruff because nits are cigar-shaped and stick to the hair shaft, rather than flake off easily; most commonly found in hair at ears and nape of neck.	Remove child's shirt. Treat scalp and neck with medicated shampoo or lotion (you may want to check with your doctor on what to get). Dry child's hair; then remove nits with a nit comb, tweezers or your fingernails. Examine each strand of hair under a bright light. If necessary, apply vinegar to child's hair to loosen nits and then comb. Change child into clean clothes.	• Advise children not to share hats, combs or other personal articles. • Check child's hair for nits daily for at least 10 days after applying medication. • Head lice do not carry disease and are more of a nuisance than a medical concern.
Herpangina (inflammation of the inside of the mouth)	Diarrhea (sometimes); high-grade fever (103°F or higher); much discomfort; many painful, distinct grayish-white ulcers on back roof of mouth and over tongue; pain when swallowing; sometimes a pink rash on trunk.	See your doctor. Plenty of non-acidic or non-carbonated fluids; soft foods. Give acetaminophen for fever and pain.	• Occurs mostly in the summer and fall in temperate climates. • Makes child miserable. • Very contagious.
Herpes simplex (stomatitis, cold sores, fever blisters)	Reduced appetite; low-grade fever; swollen, red and sometimes bleeding gums; blisters on tongue, gums, lips and around mouth; irritability.	Plenty of non-acidic or non-carbonated fluids; soft foods; acetaminophen. See doctor for antiviral ointment.	• Don't use cortisone creams. • This is a latent virus that may frequently recur.

Illness	Symptoms	Treatment	Worth Noting
Hives	Red, raised circular areas the size of a dime or quarter with red borders and pale centers; rash fades when pressed, may cover child's whole body.	Over-the-counter antihistamine; soothing compounds added to a cool bath. Cut fingernails to discourage scratching.	• Usually due to allergy. • Make list of food and other allergens to which your child was exposed in the past 24 hours. • Most common causes: pollens, insect bites, drugs, foods (especially dairy products, wheat, chocolate, pork, eggs, shellfish, berries, tomatoes and nuts). • Hives look worse than they really are; usually do not bother a child and disappear in four or five days. • No cause to worry as long as child is not wheezing or having difficulty breathing.
Impetigo (infection of the skin)	Rash, often pimple- or coin-sized, below the nose or on the buttocks; crustiness.	Ointment (prescription antibiotic, or oral antibiotic if severe). Prevent spreading by keeping covered and trimming child's fingernails to discourage scratching.	• Not highly contagious, but still wise to keep child from touching other children.
Infectious mononucleosis	Lymph nodes in neck swollen and slightly tender; low-grade fever; fatigue; sore throat.	See your doctor for diagnosis. No specific medicine for this condition. Keep child comfortable with acetaminophen for fever; adequate nutrition; lots of fluids; ice chips or popsicles for sore throat. If tonsils are swollen and obstructed, doctor may prescribe cortisone.	• May be accompanied by very large swollen tonsils. • May be confused with tonsillitis, but persists for several weeks and doesn't respond to antibiotics. • If suspected, may be confirmed by a blood test. • Contagious by exchange of saliva from child to child on contaminated objects, or during coughing or kissing.

Illness	Symptoms	Treatment	Worth Noting
Lyme disease	Flu-like symptoms; rash (which begins as a red, raised ring around a tick bite); circular, blotchy rash on trunk and extremities; swollen glands; conjunctivitis (sometimes).	Careful removal of tick *(see Tick Bites, page 21)*; antiseptic. Visit your doctor (bring tick sample along).	• Relatively rare. • Blood tests might be required to confirm diagnosis.
Measles (rubeola)	Cough; high-grade fever (103°F or higher); sensitivity to light; red eyes; a deep red rash that appears around the fourth day and begins on face, then spreads all over body.	Plenty of fluids; acetaminophen for fever; cough medicine for severe cough. Quarantine until rash is gone. Keep child out of brightly lit areas. Doctor may treat secondary complications.	• Confirmation of diagnosis by telltale white spots on inner cheeks. • You can prevent rubeola by getting your children immunized. Check with your doctor and local health department for immunization and vaccination information.
Meningitis	Convulsions; high-grade fever (103°F or higher); vomiting; increased lethargy; drowsiness; stiff neck or stiffening response to raising legs; bulging fontanel in babies; paleness; look of sickness.	Meningitis is a medical emergency. Don't attempt to treat it at home. **Take child to hospital immediately.** HIB vaccine is available to protect against Haemophilus Influenza, type B meningitis.	• Laboratory examination of spinal fluid is the only way to diagnose meningitis. • Meningitis may come on the heels of an ear infection or an upper respiratory infection. • If your child has been in contact with meningitis, **contact your doctor immediately**.
Mumps	Decreased appetite; low-grade fever; upset stomach; swollen glands beneath the earlobes two or three days later; swollen cheeks; pain when opening jaw; headache.	Bland, easy-to-digest diet; cool compresses to the neck; acetaminophen for pain and fever; isolation.	• Make sure child is vaccinated against mumps. • Contact your doctor if child becomes drowsy, persistently vomits or has a stiff neck. • One attack of mumps leads to lifetime immunity thereafter.

Illness	Symptoms	Treatment	Worth Noting
Pinworms	Restlessness; intense itching in anal or genital area; worms that look like white threads one-third of an inch long; bed-wetting; may experience abdominal cramps.	Visit your doctor (bring worms or eggs, captured by placing sticky tape around anus and using flashlight). Prescription medicine (for each family member); trimmed fingernails to discourage scratching.	• Only transmitted from person to person, not from pets or toys. • More of a nuisance than a medical concern. • Pinworms may be the cause of a recurrent inflammation of the vagina or bladder.
Pneumonia	Abdominal pain; high-grade fever (103°F or higher); chills; rapid breathing; chest pain; fast heat rate; cough; vomiting; progressive feeling of sickness.	**Seek medical attention immediately.** Fluids; mist.	• Pneumonia will resolve easily with early, aggressive treatment.
RSV (respiratory synctial virus – inflammation of the lungs)	Rapid breathing; indrawing (when you can see outline of ribs every time child breathes in); raspy cough; sore throat; paleness; tiredness; anxiety; general malaise; wheezing.	See your doctor – hospitalization may be required. Increase fluids. Small, frequent feedings.	• Watch in particular if child is becoming exhausted, or turning blue or pale around the mouth. If these symptoms are evident, **seek medical attention immediately.** • Be concerned about any lingering cough and increasingly labored breathing in infant under six months.
Reye's syndrome (inflammation of brain, liver)	High-grade fever (103°F or higher); increasing lethargy which may progress to a coma; persistent vomiting; seizures.	**Get emergency medical care.**	• Follows a viral illness. • A very serious disease. • Increased incidence of Reye's Syndrome has been associated with the use of ASA (aspirin) for fever when children have virus infections including Chicken Pox and flu.

Illness	Symptoms	Treatment	Worth Noting
Roseola	Febrile convulsions; high-grade fever (103°F or higher) that diminishes quickly with treatment and breaks on third day; faint pink rash on trunk and extremities; runny nose; slight enlargement of lymph nodes in neck. Baby does not act very ill, especially when fever goes down.	Call your doctor for fever-control advice. Acetaminophen and lukewarm baths to treat fever; plenty of fluids. Don't worry despite high fever, if child seems better when fever decreases.	• The diagnosis can't be confirmed until rash appears, usually the day after fever subsides.
Scabies (skin infection)	Intense itchiness; rash (sometimes bumpy).	Cool baths; trim finger-nails to discourage scratching; constant supply of clean under-wear; prescription cream or lotion.	• Highly contagious, but only from person to person (not from toys). • Caused by mites on or under skin.
Scarlet fever	Mid- to high-grade fever; sunburn-like rash (over face, trunk and extremities) which peels when it disappears (in five days); pallor around mouth; tonsillitis; vomiting.	Plenty of fluids; acetaminophen; bland foods. See your doctor for antibiotics.	• No more serious than strep throat. • Not very common in infants; more common in school-age children. • Contagious for 24 to 48 hours after treatment begins.
Sinusitis (sinus infection)	Cough, mainly at night; cold symptoms; pale face; puffy eyes; green or yellow thick discharge from the nose; general fatigue; low-grade fever; eye discharge.	See your doctor. Flush nose with over-the-counter saline spray. Steam from shower, vaporizer or facial steamer; extra fluids.	• A common cold that lingers for a week or more or a cold that "just won't go away" may be a sinus infection. • Recurrent sinus infections, often due to allergies, are usually due to inhalant allergens in child's bedroom. • Often overlooked because child often seems not to be very sick, just "has that tired look."

Illness	Symptoms	Treatment	Worth Noting
Strep throat	Abdominal pain; high-grade fever (103°F or higher); sore throat; red, swollen tonsils sometimes covered with white material; red patches on roof of mouth; white tongue; swollen glands; vomiting; difficulty swallowing; rash (sometimes).	Visit your doctor. Isolation (especially from other children); acetaminophen to relieve pain and fever; fluids; bland diet.	• Guard against dehydration. • Contagious for 24 to 48 hours after treatment begins. • Continue medical treatment as prescribed by doctor, even if child seems better.
Tetanus (lockjaw)	Convulsions; muscle spasms (generally jaw muscles).	Hospitalization; antibiotics.	• Highly uncommon, especially in immunized countries. • You can get your child immunized. Check with your doctor and local health department. • Can result from a severely infected wound.
Thrush	Yeast infection in baby's mouth that looks like cottage-cheese patches on inner lips, tongue, cheeks and roof of mouth; not a serious infection and seldom bothers baby.	See your doctor. Paint a prescription anti-fungal medication on patches and the rest of mouth and tongue four times a day for ten days. Often recurs, requiring a second course of treatment; often accompanied by diaper rash requiring anti-fungal ointment.	• Yeast infections in mouth and/or diaper area commonly follow antibiotic therapy because the antibiotic kills good bacteria that normally keep the yeast under control. • Giving acidophilus drops or powder (available from the pharmacy or nutrition store) while child is on antibiotic therapy can prevent yeast infection. • Thrush seldom bothers babies, but some may become irritable because of soreness in the mouth. • Thrush can be transferred to the nipples of a breast-feeding mother. If nipples are tender, pink, flaky, and itchy, it's necessary to treat mother as well as baby.

Illness	Symptoms	Treatment	Worth Noting
Tonsillitis	Sore throat; low-grade fever; slightly or very swollen glands under jaw; inflamed tonsils, often with white or yellow spots.	Plenty of liquids; vaporizer or humidifier; nose drops or oral decongestants and a nasal aspirator to relieve congestion; cough medicine if cough is severe; bland diet. Doctor may prescribe antibiotics.	• See your doctor for diagnosis. Cause may be virus or bacteria. Contagiousness, duration and treatment depend on cause. • Children between the ages of three and nine often have enlarged tonsils and adenoids. This enlargement is normal: don't confuse it with infection. White, cheesy substance on tonsils is also normal.
Urinary tract infection	Older child may complain of burning or pain when urinating; baby or toddler may show unexplained fevers, vomiting, frequent night waking, and poor growth if chronic.	See your doctor for antibiotics. Give extra fluids.	• Important to do urinalysis, but may require a urine culture. • Important not to miss because it could cause damage to kidneys if undetected and untreated.
Whooping Cough (Pertussis)	Labored breathing; low-grade fever; sneezing; watery eyes; dry cough; mucus expelled during bursts of staccato coughs, followed by long catch-up inhale.	See your doctor for antibiotics. Hospitalization for infants. Plenty of fluids; cool mist; expectorant cough syrups.	• Begins like a cold, but lingers. • Cough worsens around two weeks into the illness. • Lasts three to six weeks. • Call your doctor if symptoms persist or worsen, or if child has difficulty breathing. • You can get your child immunized against pertussis. Check with your doctor and local health department.

childhood illness record

Date   **Record here any childhood illnesses and how they were treated**

continued on next page

childhood illness record

Date   **Record here any childhood illnesses and how they were treated**

section 3

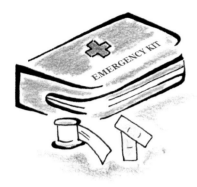

Your Child's Personal Health Journal

Table of Contents

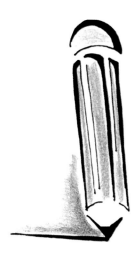

your child's personal health journal

introduction

This Personal Health Journal has been designed to help you understand your child's health and to provide a record of important health and medical information. You may need it to review it with your physician, other medical specialists and your child's teacher or caregiver.

Keep this book together with a current color photo of your child and any health insurance or hospital admission cards. You will want to keep it with you – especially when you travel.

your child's personal information

Your child's full name   Nickname

Your child's home address

Phone   Date of birth

Data on Family

Mother   Phone

                                                Cellular phone number

Father   Phone

                                                Cellular phone number

Alternate Contact   Relationship

Phone   Cellular phone number

Special Notes

emergency numbers

Ambulance

Police

Fire department

Physician's name

Hospital emergency

Dentist's name

Drugstore and phone number

(In many large urban centers, you can dial 911 for an ambulance or police and fire departments. However, this service is not available in all communities. Be sure to look in your local telephone directory or check with your local police department to find out if the 911 number operates in your community.)

Phone

Poison information center

Phone

All night drugstore and phone number

People to Contact
(in an emergency, if you are not available):

Name	Relationship	Phone Number

emergency tips

Serious injuries and emergencies should be handled by experts – know how and where to call for help. However, in some situations, prompt attention could save a life. For specific instructions, see *Sections 1 and 2, Medical Emergencies & Childhood Illnesses*.

General Procedures

choking

Hold child head-down across your arm or knee. Pat sharply between shoulders until object is coughed out. If the child is unable to cough, reach into throat with your finger to draw object forward.

burns

Smother flames with coat, rug or your own body. If you cover child quickly and completely, you will not be burned.

drowning

Pull child from water and hold with head tilted down to help water drain out. If child is not breathing, begin mouth-to-mouth resuscitation.

electric shock

If child is still part of electric circuit, don't touch him. Turn off power source if possible. If that is not possible, use dry, non-metallic object (broom, chair, etc.) to push child away.

bleeding

If blood is spurting, **act immediately**. If possible, raise injured part above heart and press hard directly on wound.

poison

If child has swallowed poison (or if you suspect he has), **call physician or the Poison Information Center immediately**.

aspirin

Although aspirin (ASA) is a commonly used pain reliever among adults, do not give it to your child without consulting your doctor first. The use of aspirin products during cases of chicken pox and flu-like viruses in children has been associated with Reye's syndrome – a potentially fatal illness. Acetaminophen products (such as Tempra and Children's Tylenol) can provide pain relief and treat fevers without the dangers of Reye's syndrome.

identification

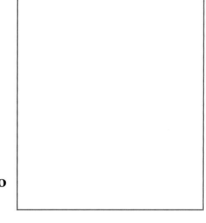

photo

It is a good idea to update your child's photo about every four to six months. *Attach a current photo to this book.*

Your child's photo

The drawings below are provided to record important identifying marks. Ask your physician for help in filling them out.

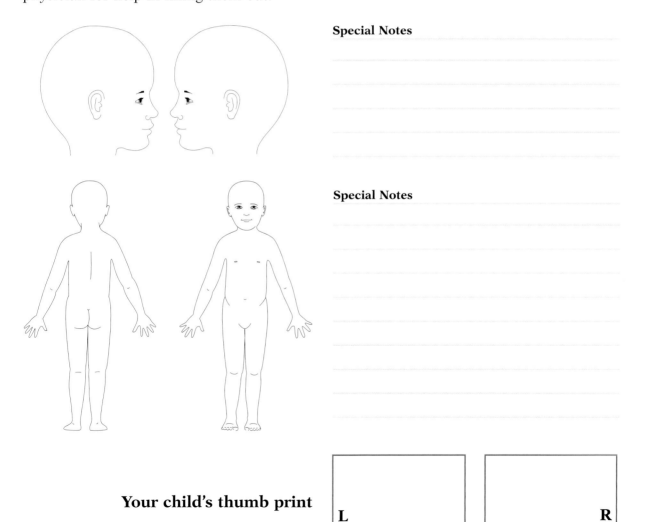

Special Notes

Special Notes

Your child's thumb print

L

R

birth history

Date .... Time ....

Place ....

Weight .... Length ....

Apgar score .... Blood type ....

Doctor in attendance ....

Comments on labor and delivery

....

....

....

....

....

Special Notes

....

....

....

....

....

....

....

immunizations

Diphtheria, tetanus, polio, pertussis (whooping cough), measles, mumps, meningitis and rubella (German measles) are serious childhood diseases. The best protection we have against them is immunization — discuss this with your doctor or health professional.

Children may experience mild side effects at the time of immunization, such as fever or a sore arm, but the benefits can far outweigh the risk of such discomforts. Serious adverse reactions to immunization are rare.

Some children should not have vaccines without a doctor being consulted:

- those who are sick right now with something more serious than a cold
- those who have had convulsions or other problems with the nervous system
- those who have had serious reactions to vaccinations before.

If you have questions about immunizations, be sure to discuss them with your physician, the immunization or public health nurse, or your community's local health department.

immunization record

(to be completed with an appropriate health professional)

Vaccine	Approx. Age of Child	Date
	(check with your doctor or local health department)	
Diphtheria, tetanus, pertussis and polio *(schedule should be recommended by your doctor)*	2 months 4 months 6 months 18 months 4-6 years (at time of school entry)	
Measles, mumps and rubella (MMR) *(schedule should be recommended by your doctor)*	12-15 months 4-6 years	
Haemophilus B (meningitis vaccine) *(schedule should be recommended by your doctor)*	2 months 4 months 6 months 18 months	
Hepatitis B vaccine *(schedule should be recommended by your doctor)*		
Chicken pox vaccine (Varicella) *(schedule should be recommended by your doctor)*		

Problems Related to Immunization   Date

tips on dealing with your doctor and other medical professionals

Doctors are often unaware of hidden factors that influence their patients' health. These factors can hinder their efforts to treat the condition. Parents often fail to provide all the information doctors need to reach a diagnosis and prescribe the appropriate treatment for their child. Good communication can help prevent these kinds of problems.

Suggestions

- Make the most of your time with your child's doctor by planning what issues you want to cover and what you want to get out of the meeting.

- Think ahead about the sort of questions your doctor will ask. Prepare yourself to provide specific details. What are your child's symptoms? When did they begin? Write it down.

- When asking questions of your doctor or medical professional, keep them simple, direct and to the point. The more specific your questions, the more likely they are to elicit useful information for you.

- Take notes or ask your doctor to write down instructions. An appointment goes by quickly and you may forget the details by the time you get home.

- Ask if you can call back and talk to someone in the office, a nurse, for example, if you have any problems or questions.

- Make sure you do not leave until you understand exactly how to administer your child's medication or treatment.

- Remember, working with your child's physician as a partner will improve the quality of your child's health care and will avoid potentially dangerous misunderstandings.

- Record any significant treatments in this journal.

child's medical history

Regular doctor appointments

Doctor	Date	Lab tests	Prescriptions	Reactions

child's medical history

Accidents, Surgeries and Illnesses

Date	Age	Doctor

Accidents, Surgeries and Illnesses - treatment and reactions

family medical history

Illness	Mother's History	Father's History
Heart disease		
Cancer		
Diabetes		
Kidney disorders		
Muscular disorders		
Cystic fibrosis		
Tay-Sachs		
Sickle cell		
Asthma		
Allergies		
Others		

allergies

Children, like adults, can have allergic reactions to foods, medicines, pets, dust and other environmental factors. It is important to keep a record of any allergic reactions your child has had.

Date	Allergy	Reaction

growth and development

Every child is unique. Each one grows and develops at his or her own pace. Many parents keep track of developmental milestones such as rolling over or taking first steps. You can record your child's growth and development in the chart below.

Milestone	Child's Age	Date
Rolls over:		
Crawls:		
Stands with support:		
Stands alone:		
Walks:		
First words:		
Other (eg. uses drinking cup for first time)		

height and weight record

Date	Age	Weight	Height

insurance information

HMO/State or Provincial Health Insurance Number:

Other Insurance Coverage:

Insurer:

Address:

Phone:

Policy number:

Other Insurance Coverage:

Insurer:

Address:

Phone:

Policy number:

**Many hospitals provide special admission cards at your first admission to the hospital.
If you receive such a card, make sure you bring it with you for every hospital visit.**

list of international medical contacts

The International Association for Medical Assistance to Travellers (IAMAT) www.sentex.net/~iamat   e-mail: iamat@sentex.net

United States
417 Center Street
Lewiston, NY
14092
716-754-4883

Canada
40 Regal Road, Guelph, ON N1K 1B5
519-836-0102 or
1287 St. Clair Ave., West, Toronto ON M6E 1B8
416-652-0137

This non-profit group publishes the IAMAT Directory, a handy guide listing the names, addresses, and phone numbers of medical centers and doctors around the world whose training meets North American or European standards.

Medic Alert

United States
2323 Colorado Avenue
Turlock, CA
95382
1-888-633-4298
www.medicalert.org./signup2.asp

Canada
2005 Sheppard Ave East, Suite 800
Toronto, Ontario
M2G 5B4
1-800-668-1507
www.medicalert.ca

This international non-profit organization was established to help people communicate vital medical information in emergencies.

Centers for Disease Control and Prevention

International Travelers' Information Line
1-800-311-3435 or www.cdc.gov

This organization provides information for travelers who need vaccine information and advice about food and water precautions when traveling.

Others

Canadian Paediatric Society
www.cps.ca   (613) 526-9397
American Academy of Pediatrics
www.aap.org   1-800-433-9016

notes

notes

notes

notes

accreditation

Medical Emergencies & Childhood Illnesses is based on the works of Dr. William Sears.

Editors: Dali Castro and Carol Lawlor

Designers: The Adlib Group and Beth Gorbet

Look for these Parent**Smart** Books at leading bookstores and other retail outlets

Joyful and Confident Parenting

This book is essential reading for every new parent. Here is the information and step-by-step advice parents need from the day their new baby joins the family.

Joyful and Confident Parenting addresses the issue of baby bonding with mom and dad as well as others in the extended family, including other caregivers. Readers will learn the steps to help build solid parent-child relationships that will last a lifetime.

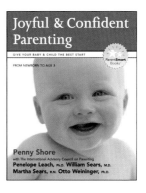

The book examines how each member of the family's parenting team can play a meaningful role in the new baby's development. The chapter entitled *Taking Stock* encourages parents to consider their own personal parenting style, the way they were raised by their parents, and how these factors will affect the way they approach the parenting of their own child.

Topics covered in *Joyful and Confident Parenting* include:

- newborn basics
- your parenting style
- baby-proofing your home
- choosing childcare
- creating a support system
- avoiding some parenting pitfalls
- how to achieve positive parenting
- building a healthy parent-child relationship

This book provides parents with the basics of joyful and confident parenting.

Positive Discipline

Some of the most challenging situations for parents and their child involve dealing with discipline issues. Starting with the basic premise that discipline starts with love, this book looks at changing discipline needs, as children go through early stages of development.

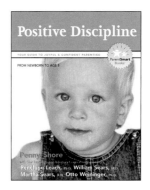

Topics covered in *Positive Discipline* include:

- how discipline techniques can affect a child's self-esteem
- the characteristics of positive discipline
- handling your own emotions and anger
- the trouble with spanking
- discipline versus punishment
- avoiding tantrums
- why you can't spoil with love
- setting appropriate limits

This book provides parents with eight practical strategies they can use to encourage cooperation from their children, and sets out easy-to-follow techniques for handling various discipline issues, including tantrums, defiance and anger. There are sections that provide guidance on dealing with discipline problems when a child is living part-time with separated or divorced parents, and on how parents can better manage their own anger, to the benefit of their children and parenting partners.

Your Baby and Child's
Growth and Development

From the moment of conception, a child's rate of growth and development is determined by a complex combination of genetic and environmental factors. This book helps parents to fully understand the factors affecting their baby's growth and development.

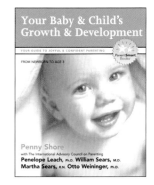

The book is organized into separate sections, each dealing with a particular phase of development, including the first six months and up to preschool. Each section looks at the factors of most concern during the particular period, including weight gain, changes in nutritional requirements, sleep patterns, increased mobility, speech and language development.

Growth and Development provides invaluable guidelines to help parents manage their baby's environment during these first vitally important years.

Topics covered in *Growth and Development* include:
- when to start baby on solid foods
- changing sleep patterns
- physical activities and feelings
- your child in play groups
- what to anticipate at each growth stage
- weight gain
- body awareness
- toddler's self-esteem
- fun and fitness

This book provides parents with an easy-to-follow guide to their baby and child's growth and development.

How Your Baby & Child Learns

Most parents want their child to have a love of learning and to do well in school. Recent research now confirms that there is much that parents can do to provide the care and stimulation which enhances learning in the first few years. *How Your Baby & Child Learns* contains information on numerous subjects, including creating a positive learning environment, a baby's early brain development and dealing with children who have special needs.

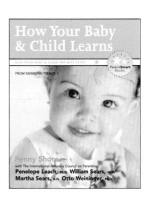

This book explores the stages of a baby's intellectual development. It provides information, as well as tips and techniques, on how parents can stimulate their child's interest in reading and how learning music also enhances mathematical abilities.

Topics covered in *How Your Baby & Child Learns* include:
- how the brain is hard-wired
- learning social responsibility
- numbers and quantitative thinking
- learning through friends
- talking to your baby
- stimulating a healthy curiosity
- talking and listening
- learning through play
- learning by pretending
- toddlers and television
- reading to your child
- music and learning

This book gives parents the information they need to enhance their child's learning opportunities.

Your Baby and Child's
Emotional and Social Development

New research gives us a better understanding of how babies develop emotionally and socially. This book will give parents new insights into these important developmental processes and things they can do to enhance the long term well-being and feelings of security in their child.

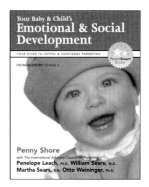

Topics covered in *Emotional and Social Development* include:

- ten strategies for your child's healthy emotional development
- baby's feelings
- what it means when babies cry
- the importance of a baby's gaze
- the child-friendly environment
- the five senses
- toddler socializing
- the parent partnership
- enriching the bond

Readers will learn the timing of emotional development, from the child's initial bonding with the parents, to relating to others outside of the immediate family.

This book is must reading for every parent who is concerned with the emotional and social well-being of their child.

The International Advisory Council on Parenting

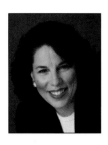

Penny Shore
Created the *ParentSmart Books* and is President of The Parent Kit Corporation. She was Vice President, Product Development for Hume Publishing, and a management consultant with degrees in psychology and gerontology. An expert on the development of home study programs on a variety of topics, Ms. Shore is a parenting educator and an advocate for effective parenting.

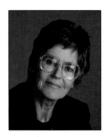

Penelope Leach, Ph.D.
Was educated at Cambridge University, London School of Economics and University of London, where she received her Ph.D. in psychology. She is a renowned author of many books, including *Your Baby and Child* and *Your Growing Child*, fellow of the British Psychological Society, past President of the Child Development Society and acknowledged international expert on the effects of parents' different child-rearing styles on children.

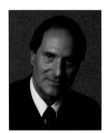

William Sears, M.D.
Regarded as one of North America's leading pediatricians, is a medical and parenting consultant to several magazines and organizations, and a frequent guest on television shows. Dr. Sears received his pediatric training at Harvard Medical School's Children's Hospital and Toronto's Hospital for Sick Children. He is the author of many books on parenting, including *The Baby Book* and *The Discipline Book*.

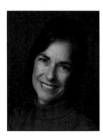

Martha Sears, R.N.
Is a registered pediatric nurse and co-author, with her husband, William Sears, of many books on parenting, including *Parenting the Fussy Baby and the High-Need Child.* In addition to being a regular contributor to several national magazines for parents, she has appeared on more than a hundred television shows and is a popular speaker at parents' organizations across North America.

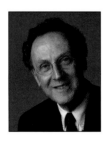

Otto Weininger, Ph.D.
Served for 15 years as chairman of the Early Childhood Program at the University of Toronto, where he received his Ph.D. in psychology. He is the author of several books including *Time In* and former editor of *The International Journal of Early Childhood Education*. He is a host and frequent guest on radio and television programs around the world, sharing his expertise on children's education, play, learning and relationships.

YOUR PARENTING JOURNAL

Date   **Comments**

YOUR PARENTING JOURNAL

Date   **Comments**

YOUR PARENTING JOURNAL

Date   **Comments**

YOUR PARENTING JOURNAL

Date

Comments

YOUR PARENTING JOURNAL

Date

Comments

YOUR PARENTING JOURNAL

Date   **Comments**

YOUR PARENTING JOURNAL

Date   **Comments**

index